Hair Secrets

How To Stop Hair Loss
&
Regrow Your Hair Faster
Naturally!

Engy Khalil

Table of Contents

IMPORTANT COPYRIGHT AND LEGAL NOTICE:

Disclaimer And Copyright Notification

The book Hair Secrets: How to Stop Hair Loss & Regrow Your Hair Faster Naturally! is intended to provide helpful information and guidance to people who seek to improve their health. It discusses the numerous reasons and causes of hair loss in women and provides simple methods to combat the situation and grow their hair again. This e-book is intended for educational purposes only and addresses the health issues that cause hair loss. We do not provide guarantee for the efficacy or safety of any of the treatment options listed here. Readers are requested to consult their general physicians before approaching natural and artificial methods of treatment and remedies for hair loss.

How to Use This Guide

First i want to thank you for buying my program, everything you will read in this book comes from years of a hard work and many research as well as experience with thousands of my clients for this techniques. These techniques worked well for me and all my clients, they noticed changes in their hair as well as their whole health.

To get great results from this program, you should read carefully all the Book from A to Z, don't skip any chapter or word as you will find ideas and solutions between the lines.

Important Notes: For the natural Remedies please before trying any of this you must test a small patch to ensure you don't have any allergic to the ingredients.

Also if you have scalp scratches, scalp acne or inflammation in your scalp treat these first then try the Remedies.

If you are pregnant don't try any of this recipes and remedies before consulting your doctor.

If you have any allergies to some food that are in the natural recipes that means if you apply it to your scalp, you will get the same allergies in scalp, the solution is to replace it with another one

What You Will Learn in "Hair Secrets!"

As a busy working woman with many responsibilities, you may not have all the time in the world to tend to your tresses. Hair health and appearance is a common worry that plagues many women. Ranging from hair fall, dandruff, and dryness, weak and brittle hair can cause you a lot of unwanted stress.

If you have been exposed to the sun, pollutants and haven't had time to improve your lifestyle, now is your chance. This book has been designed to help you improve your overall approach to hair care and transform the way you care for your skin.

With the right foods entering your system, you can achieve strength and flexibility in your hair from within. The right nutrients can improve your tresses by providing resilience, shine and strength to deal with the everyday worries of work and home.

Apart from eating the right foods, exercising regularly can have a surprising effect on your hair. By boosting blood circulation and ensuring a regular endorphin rush, you can bring down the stress levels in your body and allow your scalp to remain healthy.

With rich oxygenated blood filled with nutritional goodness reaching your hair roots every day, your hair care regime is significantly shortened. No longer do you need expensive hair masks, conditioners and serums to keep them soft, shiny and strong.

Another way you can definitely improve your hair health is to align your needs to natural solutions. While off the rack hair products make tall promises, they only work from the outside. Filled with

chemicals and undesirable toxins, these expensive products may make your hair look shiny from the outside but only damage the natural build of your tresses.

This is why it is best to turn to natural remedies and therapies to nurture your hair. This book also highlights a number of natural ways through which you can strengthen your hair and make it shinier, longer and more resistant to the everyday wear and tear caused by pollution, dust, grime and UV rays.

Introducing – Your Hair!

How Does Your Hair Grow?

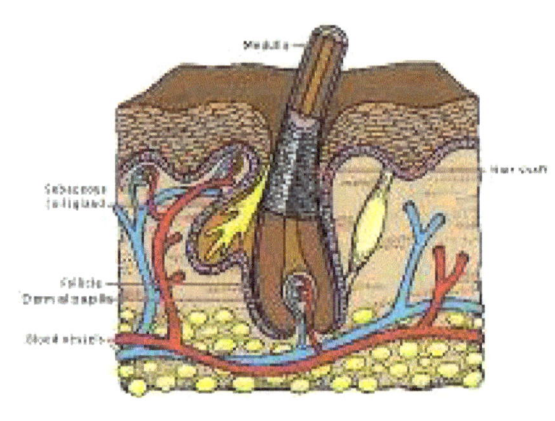

Apart from appearance and physical protection of the scalp, your hair has many purposes and benefits. Being more complex than imagined, hair is also essential in transmitting sensory information and to create gender distinction and identification.

Even in the fetal stage, hair follicles are useful. By the 22nd week, all hair follicles in the body are already formed. At this stage, about five million hair follicles are formed on the body.

About one million hair follicles are found in the head, with about 100,000 formed on your scalp. It is estimated to be the largest number of follicles an average human has.

It is interesting to note that you do not generate or produce new hair follicles in your life. Another interesting thing you may have noticed about hair is that the general density of your scalp hair decreases as you grow into an adult. This need not indicate a reduction in the number of hair follicles, rather a spread out of the follicles since your scalp expands as your body grows.

What is it Composed of?

The human hair is comprised of four distinct parts i.e. the follicle, cortex, cuticle and medulla.

However, the follicle itself is made of many other parts. It is interesting to note that hair follicles are among the only two places in an adult human where stem cells are available.

On an average, your hair grows about six inches in a year and dies in the next four years. Your hair can also be divided into the follicle and shaft, the latter being visible over the scalp.

Hair follicle

The hair follicle can be defined as a tunnel like portion of the epidermal layer of the skin that extends all the way into the dermis. The structure of the hair follicle includes multiple layers with unique and separate functions. The base of your hair follicle is known as the papilla and contains blood capillaries that nourish your scalp and hair. The living part in your hair strands, known as the bulb, is located at the bottom of the scalp and surrounds the papilla.

The cells existing in the bulb divide every 1–3 days and are significantly faster than other cells in your body. It is this splitting of cells, which results in hair growth, and can vary from person to person.

The hair follicle is surrounded by inner sheath and outer sheath that protect and allow the hair shaft or strand to grow. The inner sheath ends below the oil glands, also known as the sebaceous gland or apocrine glands. The outer sheath on the other hand continues till the gland itself.

Arrector pili

A muscle named arrector pili is attached to a fibrous layer surrounding the bottom sheath at the lower part of the gland. When this muscle contracts; it results in the hair strands to stand up. Arrectores pilorum (plural) are generally made of minute muscle fibers. The contraction of these muscles is involuntary and is often induced by cold weather. That is why you often experience goosebumps in cold weather or even air conditioned environments.

Sebaceous glands

The same function commands the sebaceous glands to secrete oil and protect hair strands. The sebaceous gland is very important to maintain and protect hair health as it produces sebum, a substance that is known to condition your skin and hair.

When you reach puberty, your body starts producing more sebum and the production slowly reduces as your age. In fact, women are known to produce far less amounts of sebum in their body than men of the same age.

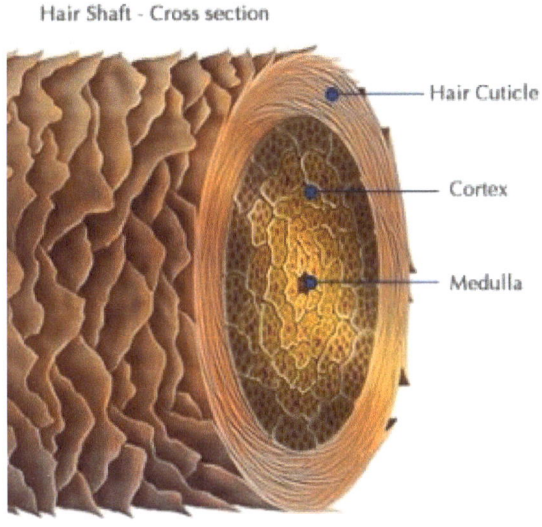

Illustration 1: Hair shafts

Hair shafts

Hair shafts are made of hard proteins known as keratin and can be divided into three distinct layers. The protein found in your hair is actually dead, making hair a non-living yet growing part of your body. The three parts of the hair shaft include the medulla, cortex and cuticle that are responsible for many distinctions in hair including color, strength, pigmentation, and so on.

Medulla: The medulla or medullary canal is located inside the cortex of the hair shaft and contains only air. Despite being an integral part of the hair shaft, medulla does not have any effect or influence on the properties or traits of human hair.

Cortex: The cortex surrounds the medullary canal and is situated inside the cuticle. Unlike medulla that does not have any correlation with the traits of human hair; the cortex is responsible for the weight, width and visual appearance of the hair.
It comprised of multiple braided fibers with pigments of red, yellow, brown and black.

The relative ratios of these pigments determine your hair color. This layer of the hair shaft is also responsible for many other traits of human hair including, thickness, straightness, and toughness, and is mainly made of water and protein.

Cuticle: While the cortex and medulla are found underneath the scalp, the cuticle is the protective layer found on the outside. The cuticle consists of keratin, a hard non–living protein and surrounds every strand of hair.

While the cortex is responsible for the waviness, straightness and strength of the hair, the cuticle determines the sheen. Well–maintained cuticles can reflect light effectively and give your hair a healthy and natural shine.

The cuticle is mainly made of scales that grow and point towards the tips and can include anywhere between five and 12 layers. It is mainly translucent and is not the main source of hair color. The cuticle protects the cortex layer inside and brings out the color based on its color pigment composition.

The Phases Of Hair Growth Cycle

Hair follicles function with repeated cycles of growth and each cycle can be broken down into three distinct phases – Anagen, Catagen and Telogen. Every single strand of hair on your scalp undergoes these three phases in each cycle and is completely independent of the other strands of hair on your scalp.

Anagen phase

This phase is also called the active phase or the growth phase of your hair. At least 85 percent of all the strands of hair on the scalp are in this stage at any given time.

The anagen phase is much longer than you might expect and runs anywhere between two and six years.

Hair roughly grows 10 centimeters every year on an average while the rate of growth can vary from person to person. In any case, the

total length of a single strand of hair is unlikely to grow after reaching the length of one meter. During this stage, the cells in the hair root are dividing at a rapid pace and new hair is formed quickly. The newly formed hair pushes the club hair up and out of the follicle.

In simple terms, club hair can be defined as specific strands of hair that have already passed the anagen phase. During this phase, your hair can grow about one centimeter every 28 days and remains active for several years.

Some people find it easier to grow their hair longer than others because of their lengthened active growth phase. The duration of the active phase of growth can decide how long your hair can be grown. The hair on your arms, legs, eyebrows and eyelashes have very short spurts of growth, lasting between 30 to 45 days. This is the reason why your body hair is never as long as your scalp.

Catagen phase

This phase is a transitional period between the growth and resting. Roughly three percent of your scalp hair is at this stage at a time, lasting between two and three weeks at a time. After the growth stops, the sheath in the outer root shrinks, attaching itself to the root of your hair. This process is known as the formation of the club hair. During this phase, the hair follicle shrinks to 1/6th of its normal length and lower part of the hair is destroyed. The catagen phase also sees the breakage of dermal papilla, resting below on the surface of the scalp.

Telogen phase

The Telogen phase is known as the resting phase. Roughly six to eight percent of all the hair on your scalp is at this stage at the same time. The Telogen phase lasts for about 100 days on the scalp. For body hair like eyelashes, eyebrows, arms and legs, the phase is much longer.

During the Telogen phase, hair follicles are at complete rest while the club hair is formed completely.

When you pull out a hair at this stage, you will notice a dry, hard and solid white material at its root. The Telogen phase also accounts for the normal hair fall. Roughly 25 to 100 strands of hair that are in this phase are shed every day and this is no reason for alarm.

During the Telogen phase, your hair stops growing, but remains attached to your hair follicle. The dermal papilla is also in place during the resting phase. When the Telogen phase approaches its end, a new anagen phase begins the next cycle.

The base of your hair follicle and dermal papilla rejoin and a new hair begins to form and grow. If the old hair in the same place has not already been shed, the new growing hair pushes it out, beginning the next growth cycle.

Main Functions of Human Hair

One of the primary functions of human hair is to protect your body and regulate temperature.

With over five million hair follicles distributed throughout your body and scalp, your body works hard to maintain the right temperatures. While your body hair is mainly to control these temperatures, the hair on your scalp is to protect your skull.

Being one of the most important parts of your body, your scalp requires additional protection from the sun. It is also one of the few body parts that are exposed to maximum sunlight. This is why greater protection is required to ward off heat and radiations. With varying thicknesses, textures, lengths and properties, **human hair serves a number of purposes as listed below:**

1- Hair protects your scalp from external elements like sun damage and drying. It also protects your scalp from chapping from extreme wind and prevents dirt and dust from settling on your skin.

For example: If you expose to the sun's rays in summer or use hair dryer (blow-dry) on thinning hair that is mean your scalp and follicles is very easy to damage and burn from the hot air. so hair is serving as a physical barrier between your skin and the external atmosphere and trapping warm air between the hair and skin. The insulation purposes of hair are useful in both cold and warm temperatures and ensure proper temperature regulation in your body.

2- The importance of hair for all women, is that it can attract attention. Hair increase self-confidence of women and identify facial features. Sometimes the woman is not beautiful enough but she has a long lusters hair, She usually use her beautiful hair to serve as a compensation for ordinary face.

Evident From The Above, It Is Very Important To Maintain And Protect Your Hair Not Only For The Outer Shape But Also For Healthy Body And Skin.

What Causes Hair Loss?

Hair loss is completely normal. On a daily basis when you are showering, combing or styling your hair, it is completely normal to expect some amount of hair fall. Losing about 50–100 strands of hair per day is completely normal.

However, excessive hair loss can cause alarm as it more often a sign of an underlying problem and while it seems more frequent in men, it can also affect women.

If you are noticing significant hair fall and thinning, the underlying cause could be one of the following. In any case, it is best to pay a visit to your trusted dermatologist for help.

There are several factors which may lead to hair loss and thinning hair.

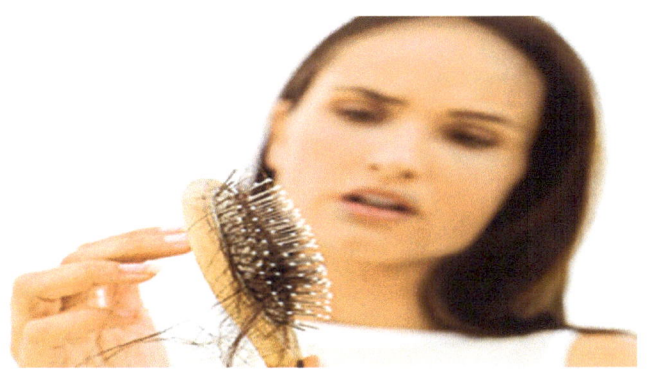

Stress

Pollution

Genetic hair loss

Female pattern baldness

Thyroid disease

Lupus

PCOS And Imbalance Hormone

Improper diet

Iron deficiency

Impulse control disorder

Alopecia Areata

Aging

Medication

Excessive styling

Skin conditions

Parasites

Product Build-up

Hair Tension

Rapid weight-loss

In order to know what are exactly the causes of hair loss and thinning hair you need to look to your body health and scalp as healthy hair comes only from healthy body and scalp. It is important to read this chapter carefully that can help every woman to know problems and it may serve as a cautionary as to know what should to do and what should to avoid.

Stress

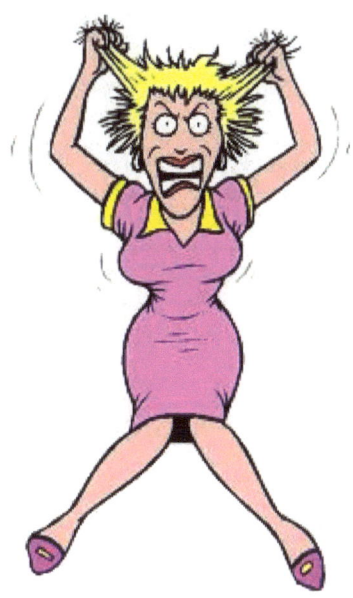

It comes as no surprise that stress can lead to hair fall. Everyday stress or extreme stress due to a one off event can trigger negative changes in your body, including hair loss. Apart from regular stress, any event or experience that causes emotional or physical trauma can lead to hair loss. This can include anything from a severe illness, surgery, accident, leading to temporary hair loss.

During a stressful event, your hair cycle undergoes a shock when most of your hair begins the shedding phase. In such cases, hair loss is apparently only after about 3-6 months. However, with the right diet and care for you mental and physical health, you can nurse your hair back to life as your body continues to recover and strengthen.

The scientific term for this event is called Telogen effluvium, a phenomenon commonly observed after a major surgery, accident, illness, pregnancy or other events that cause extreme amounts of stress. During this phase, your hair shifts from its growing phase to the shedding phase much quicker than normal. While there are no tests to definitely identify Telogen effluvium, you can speak to your doctor about your hair loss systems and determine the functioning of the hair growth cycle.

If the cause for Telogen effluvium is stress related, taking direct and indirect measures to reduce anxiety can benefit your hair.
find unique ways to beat stress, whether it is taking up a new hobby, speaking to a therapist, working out or even meditating as this will directly influence the way your body recovers from stress. I tried this

before and i got very good results.

Pollution

Pollution is a major reason behind the general depreciating health of women, even causing hair loss in some. Exposure to hot weather, smoke, and everyday pollution can have a drastic impact on your hair as chemicals and industrial pollutants affect its strength and integrity. What makes it interesting is that even those who do not spend much time outdoors are at risk of pollution induced hair loss.

If you work from home or indoors for long durations of the day, you may think yourself safer than others in terms of exposure to pollution. However, you will be wrong to assume so.

There are several pollutants in your home or office that can affect the quality of your hair. Anything ranging from cigarette smoke to common dust can influence hair loss.

Cigarette smoke contains carcinogens that can easily damage your hair while the carbon content in regular smoke can damage your hair follicles. Even if nobody in your vicinity is a smoker, you are at risk through common dust that contains microorganisms that lead to scaling and itching on your scalp. These changes are generally too minute to observe, but

when left unchecked, can lead to serious problems.

In other rare cases, hair loss can be caused by pollution through food.

Frequent consumption of preservative rich foods like junk food,

packaged dinners and other processed items can introduce several

undesirable chemicals into your body, causing a different type of

pollution.

In many cases, people have reported that switching to organic and

more natural sources of food has significantly reduced hair fall. There

is merit in avoiding fast food and other chemical filled products.

Genetic Hair Loss

Genetic or hereditary hair loss is known as androgenetic alopecia and

is one of the most common causes for female hair loss. The gene

causing this form of hair fall can be inherited from either the mother

or the father's family. However, if both parents have this form of hair

loss, the chances of you facing genetic hair fall is much higher.

Some of the most common symptoms of hereditary hair loss include

hair thinning behind bangs and crown. Even some young women in their 20s are known to develop this form of hair loss and they can become vulnerable to severe baldness if not treated immediately. Sometimes, the hair loss caused by genetics can diffuse and spread to the entire scalp.

You can slow down the hair loss with the right treatment as prescribed by your dermatologist. A common diagnosis method to determine genetic hair loss is to examine the pattern and test the hair follicles for signs of damage. Also the natural hair remedies are very effective for this cases.

Female Pattern Baldness

When defined in simple terms, baldness occurs when your hair falls out, but does not replace itself. While this phenomenon is very common amongst men, female pattern baldness is not well understood. It can be caused because of a number of reasons ranging from genetics, hormonal imbalances, aging, or menopause. Symptoms of female pattern baldness are very different from male pattern baldness as the front hairline remains intact. However, hair loss and thinning most commonly occurs on the crown and top of the scalp and begins widening through the center.

Baldness in women rarely leads to complete balding as with men and only reaches as far as significant thinning and bald spots. Other symptoms of female pattern baldness are sores and itching on the scalp that are generally not obvious on sight.

In most cases, female pattern baldness can be treated when checked on time and hair loss can be minimized.

Thyroid Disease

Thyroid disease or hypothyroidism affects millions of people all over the world; a significant number of them are women. The thyroid hormone is responsible for a number of functions including heart rate, metabolism and mood. It is also responsible for the way your body utilizes oxygen and energy to the growth and strength of your skin, nails and hair.

When your body does not produce enough thyroid hormones because of an under-active thyroid, it is known as hypothyroidism. On the other hand, if your body produces too much thyroid, you are said to have hyperthyroidism i.e. an overactive thyroid. Any imbalance in the production of thyroid can lead to hair loss.

In cases of hyperthyroidism, some of the most common symptoms include sudden weight loss, irritability, nervousness, heart palpitations, and weakness in muscles, damage skin, and sudden change in the appearance of your eyes, diarrhea, hair loss, and sudden increase in metabolism.

With the right medication to treat the underlying problem of hair loss like too much or too little of the thyroid hormone, you can reduce hair fall and improve its health and appearance.

Lupus

A common chronic autoimmune disease, lupus affects millions of people around the world. The main problem caused by this disease is that your own immune system begins attacking healthy tissues in your body. Lupus mainly strikes women in their childbearing years and can cause a plethora of side effects including hair loss, if not treated at the right time.

Some of the most telltale signs of lupus include headache, swollen or painful joints, oral ulcers and fatigue. In some cases, women are known to develop rashes across the nose bridge and tend to feel very sensitive when exposed to sunlight.

These rashes are often in the shape of a butterfly owing to its location. Other symptoms of lupus include swelling in the hands and feet, anemia, fever, chest pain and hair loss. Hair fall in particular can vary from person to person as lupus causes mild to extreme amounts of hair loss. They can also accompany patching or rashes on the scalp. The condition lupus is often called the imitator as these symptoms are also found in many other health conditions, making lupus more difficult to diagnose and pinpoint.

Blood tests, tissue analyses and joint examinations are common tools used to determine lupus. If you are experiencing hair loss along with fatigue, joint pain and other related symptoms, it is wise to visit a rheumatologist immediately. Apart from oral medication, lupus can also be treated with topical creams and ointments.

PCOS And Imbalance Hormone

Polycystic ovarian syndrome affects one out of four women around the world is a surprisingly common health condition. This condition is found in women and can start as early as the age of eleven. PCOS is normally caused by hormonal imbalances that lead to your ovaries producing an excess of male hormones and can often lead to infertility. Some of the most common symptoms of polycystic ovarian syndrome include acne, facial hair growth, irregular periods, and ovarian cysts.

Apart from an increase in facial hair growth, you may also notice excessive hair loss from your scalp.

PCOS can be diagnosed with a simple blood test for testosterone levels and sonar x-ray and can be controlled by Surgical or some medications that block or reduce the production of male hormones in women.

Improper Diet

Vitamin supplements and medication can affect your hair growth. In fact, too much vitamin A can actually lead to hair fall. Fortunately, this process is easily reversible. Ensure that you stop consuming vitamin A supplements until it completely leaves your body and wait for your hair to grow back normally.

Speak to your doctor on reducing your supplement intake and

choosing natural food sources instead. A deficiency of vitamin B can also lead to hair loss. However like vitamin A, this problem is treatable and reversible.

Ensure that you find natural sources of vitamin B through non-citrus fruits, meat, fish and starch rich vegetables. You can also source healthy fats from nuts and avocados to improve the strength and texture of your hair.

Additionally, lack of protein in your diet can also lead to hair loss. If you don't source enough protein, your body starts rationing the available nutrition and shuts down hair growth. This change is visible only after a few months of the drop in, consumptions. Apart from health reasons, it is also important to consume adequate amounts of healthy protein through lean meats, low fat dairy products and fish.

Iron Deficiency

Women who do not consume enough iron rich foods or experience heavy menstrual cycles are at a greater risk of iron deficiency. This condition occurs when your blood does not have enough red blood cells. As you may already know, red blood cells are essential to transport oxygen throughout your body and deliver it to organs, tissues and living cells. This oxygen gives you enough energy to function properly.

When you have iron deficiency, you could experience paleness in skin, fatigue, weakness, headaches, cold extremities, hair loss and loss of focus. Even the most minor of physical exertions could leave you tired and short of breath. Ask your doctor about taking iron supplement.

Hair fall caused by iron deficiency can be easily countered without treatment by simply improving your diet. Include iron rich foods like leafy greens, cereals, beef liver, fish, beef, and beans. When paired with foods in vitamin C, you can improve your body's capacity to absorb iron. Apart from natural foods, you can also opt for doctor-recommended iron supplements.

Impulse Control Disorder:

Impulse control disorder, also known as Trichotillomania, is a condition that causes people to pull their hair out. This disorder is similar to a compulsion and forces the person to constantly play with their hair or pull on them.

Irrespective of the underlying causes of the condition, this constant pulling can strip your scalp of its protector. Trichotillomania is four times more common in women compared to men and can begin before the age of seventeen.

Behavioral modification therapy are the best way to control hair loss by eliminating the disorder from its root.

Alopecia Areata:

Alopecia Areata is one of the most common auto immune diseases where in your immune system attacks your hair follicles. Affecting millions of people worldwide, this disease occurs equally in both men and women. While the actual cause of the condition is depression or psychological trauma and sometimes the reasons are unknown, it is believed to be triggered by an existing or previous illness and/or stress.

Alopecia Areata can occur in three main forms. One of the most common symptoms of this form of hair loss is the appearance of smooth round bald patches on your legs, eyebrows or scalp. If you experience complete hair loss on your scalp, the condition is called alopecia totalis, while the loss of complete body hair is known as alopecia universalis. Tingling or irritation has also been noticed in affected areas.

Your doctor runs the diagnoses by observing the hair loss patterns and search for the percentage of iron in your blood. It is usually treated with a combination of medication and stress reducing measures.

Aging:

It is very common to notice hair loss after menopause for women over the age of 50. Most women do know what is the reason of this, hair fall in this age stage because the estrogen hormone level is decreased.

If you are in your 45s or 60s and are experiencing hair loss due to aging, it is best to avoid any chemical hair products.

Instead you can simply style your hair in a manner that conceals the patches and use Microfiber Keratin it is excellent to cover thinning or bald area.

Visit http://fasterhair.net/microfiberkeratin to find Microfiber Keratin

Medication:

There are certain medications that cause hair loss. Some of the most common ones include high Blood Pressure drugs and blood thinners. Other drugs and medications that can lead to hair loss include anti depressants, gout, bipolar conditions medications it can cause thyroid problems which lead to hair loss, anti inflammatory drugs, as well as medicines for skin conditions like acne capsules and rheumatic problems.

Anabolic steroids can also lead to hair thinning and is commonly consumed by bodybuilders and athletes. These steroids are known to have an impact on your body and can lead to the development of PCOS by increasing the production of testosterone and other male hormones in your body. Stop taking this medications as possible.

Chemotherapy:

Being a common form of treatment for cancer, chemotherapy can lead to excessive or even complete hair loss. It works on destroying cancer cells that are prone to divide quickly. Apart from destroying affected cells, the treatment also destroys other rapidly dividing cells found in your hair follicles. This is why most cancer patients experience a sudden loss of hair. In most cases, your hair grows back after the treatment has been completely stopped. However, there are chances that the hair will turn out to be of a different color or texture. Owing to the noticeable hair loss, even your scalp skin becomes sensitive and irritated.

One way of dealing with hair thinning and fallout during chemotherapy is to cut it very short or shave it completely. Despite being a drastic step, this has been proven to be easier for for men and women to handle as they don't notice a sudden hair loss.

If you are undergoing chemotherapy and are experiencing hair loss, there are a few steps you can follow to protect your hair from falling. It is ideal to switch to a gentle shampoo like organic or baby shampoo, this shampoos are free from harsh chemicals. Instead of using blow dryers or styling appliances, pat your hair dry or air dry it completely.

Switch to a soft brush and avoid perming or coloring your hair. You can replace hair dyes by natural henna, it is chemical free and strengthening thinning hair.

Use additional protection for your exposed scalp by wearing scarves or hats or human hair wigs.

Excessive Styling:

This is an unsurprising cause of hair fall. With the advent of chemical rich shampoos, hair dyes and other products, hair loss is an expected result.

Owing to excessive dyeing, styling and shampooing, your hair will face a lot more damage than before, as this products harm hair follicles, hair cuticle, and also makes the scalp very sensitive. As well as the chemical content in the dye and shampoos paired with the heat emanating from hair dryers and straightening or curling machines, your hair becomes weaker and eventually falls out.

In most cases, the common cause for hair loss is the combination of keratin treatment, artificial coloring and regular blow drying.

External damage caused by styling can lead to breakage and weakening of hair and compromise its strength, resilience and flexibility.

To prevent damage caused by excessive styling, it is wise to stay away from appliances that cause overheating in your hair, whether you are straightening, curling or drying your hair.

Set your hair dryer on cool or low settings and avoid using flat irons as much as possible.

If you are insisting on using hair dyes, avoid choosing colors that are more than 1-2 shades from your original color.

The more change in the hair dye, the more chemicals you need to complete the process. This exposure to heat and chemicals will definitely lead your hair to break easily.

It is also a good idea to comb your hair immediately after you apply hair gel or spray as they are more prone to breakage after they set.

Skin Conditions:

If your scalp is infected or otherwise unhealthy, it can become difficult to grow hair. Inflammation caused by skin conditions can lead to an excess of hair loss and some of the most common problems associated with scalp skin include fungal infections like ringworm, psoriasis, and dandruff (seborrheic dermatitis).

The most common symptoms for these skin conditions include yellowish scales, greasy scalp, increased shedding. This could be the result of hormonal changes, excessive oil content in the skin or the yeast Malassezia. Psoriasis is an auto immune disease that causes an excessive turnover of skin cells and produces white scales on your scalp. When pulled, they often bleed.

In cases of ringworm or other fungal infections, you could notice red patches on your scalp. Although these patches may diffuse over time, you could contract it through touching an infected animal or person.

A thorough physical examination of your scalp can determine the type of skin condition that is causing the hair loss. In terms of infections, fungal cultures and biopsies are most common. Medicated shampoos, anti-fungal natural recipes and/or creams and oral medications are commonly prescribed for ringworm and psoriasis.

Parasites

Parasites can also cause hair loss and have devastating effects on hair, parasites are objects live inside the intestines and is involved in everything you eat. Parasites can pick up from pets like dogs and cats, eating uncooked food like meat and shellfish, eating pork, during Intimacy from person to another and Bug bites as parasites can introduce into bloodstream.

To avoid parasites infection you should wash your hands before taking your meal.

Also it is very important to trim your nails regularly every week because the parasites live under nails, also brushing your nails with a clean brush everyday and cook meat and shellfish well.

Symptoms are pallor, fatigue itching around the anus and colic especially after eaten.

If you have this symptoms you should visit a doctor and do stool analysis. The treatments is available you can get rid of it very fast.

Product Build-Up

Dirts, sebum, sweat, hair products and oils clog scalp pores which lead to hair loss, slow growing and also hair breakage.

You should to use a clarifying shampoo one time a month or at least one time every 2 months, this will eliminate and help get rid the hair of dirt, sebum, and debris from harsh chemicals and toxins that product build up.

if you do not like to use clarifying shampoo apple cider vinegar rinse is the best alternative. Honestly i love to use apple cider vinegar more than clarifying shampoo because clarifying shampoo makes my hair so dry.

Hair Tension

Hair tension is pulling hair very tightly, it happens when you wear braids or buns or ponytails or wear clip or glue hair extension, too much hair tension causes thinning hair and bald area in the front of hair line and the crown area of the head which known as traction alopecia, it causes the induce follicular inflammatory, some women noticed a little bumps around the hair line and scalp pain.

The best solution to grow this areas is to stop tightly and pull your hair back at all.

The second thing is to massage this thinning area everyday before bed at least 5 minutes, if the pain and the bumps are still existing, it is important to pay a visit to the dermatologist for help.

The third important thing is to try to use essential hair vitamins.

Rapid Weight-Loss

Rapid weight loss is no less than a physical trauma for your hair. Though weight loss may be good for you, dramatic weight loss most certainly is not. Apart from taxing your metabolism and burning out the lean muscles, rapid weight loss also damages your scalp and follicles.

Rapid weight–loss is triggered by crash dieting or starvation – your body is exhausted for energy and only focuses on vital functions like working your heart and brain. Result? You're thinner and so is your hair!

Further, hair is primarily made up of proteins. Lack of a balanced diet robs your body of its protein
reserves and the body expends little or none of it on hair.

Aim for healthy weight loss, not more than two or three pounds a week. Ensure your daily consumption of protein doesn't fall below 46 grams. If your crash diet has in fact shocked your body, the hair loss will typically continue for six months , after which the body will resume normal function.

Hair Management During Pregnancy

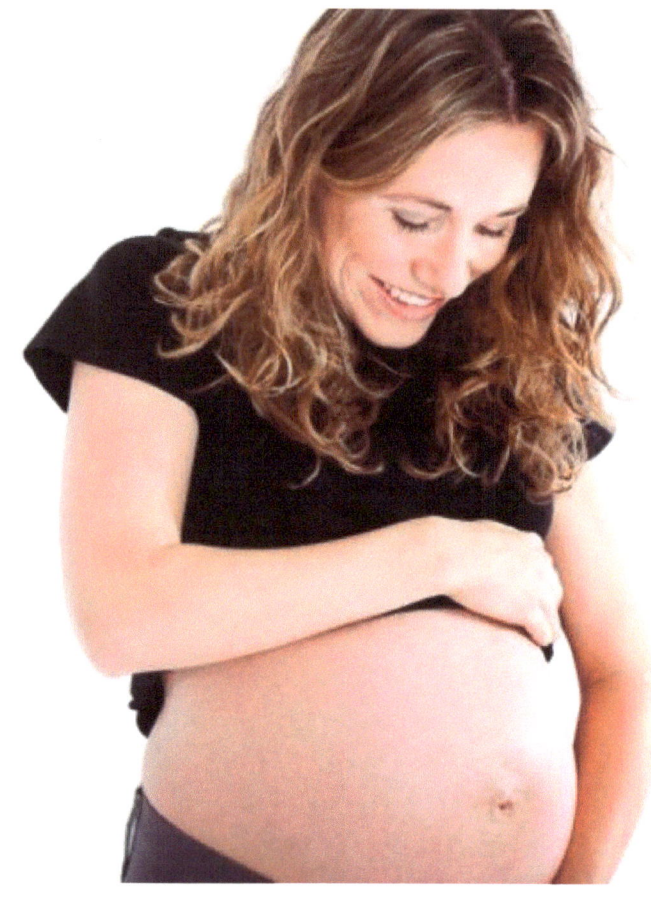

Managing your hair during pregnancy can be a tricky proposition as prescription medication is not always ideal. The following sections discuss numerous options that will help in taking care of your hair during pregnancy without having to turn to medication.

One of the most important steps you should take as a new mother is maintaining a healthy diet even after childbirth. It is important to understand that everything you eat has a direct influence on your hair and skin. Ensure that you eat as many raw fruits and vegetables as well as greens to get all the right vitamins and minerals. Turn to organic cosmetics like shampoos and conditioners instead of chemical ones as they are gentler on your hair. In many women, pregnancy has been known to change the texture of hair, making it more important to keep it moisturized and nourished. Avoid using excess shampoo or blow drying your hair too frequently. Choose protein rich shampoos that naturally add volume to your hair and avoid the use of styling appliances that damage.

This Is Just A Sample Of The Book "How Grow Secrets" To Get The Complete Version Please Visit:

Hairgrowsecret.Com

www.ingramcontent.com/pod-product-compliance
Lightning Source LLC
Chambersburg PA
CBHW041523280526
45792CB00004B/1364